THE
HCG
DIET
SYSTEM

A PHASE-BY-PHASE
BLUEPRINT FOR **SUCCESS**

The HCG Diet System -
A Phase-By-Phase Blueprint for Success

Published by

Body Confidence Bookshelf

Contact info:

KRE Book Group
PO Box 121135
Nashville, TN 37212

Table of Contents

Introduction 5

Chapter 1

HCG Diet: What Is It?.. 7
    The HCG Program In General 8
    HCG: Where It Comes From.. 9
    The Dilemma Of Fat: The Good And The Bad.......................... 10
        When It Is Good.. 10
        When It Is Bad 11
    Why Other Diet Programs Fail?.. 12
        Muscle Tissue Loss 12
        Intolerable Starvation 13
        Water Retention Loss 13
        Elaborate Exercise Programs... 14
    Why The HCG Diet Program Will Succeed 15

Chapter 2

The HCG Diet Plan: A Phase-By-Phase Approach..................... 17
    Phase One: Prepping Your Body 18
    Phase Two: Starting The Low Calorie Diet 19
    Phase Three: Entering The Maintenance Stage 22
    Re-entering The Cycle 23
    Enjoying Permanent Changes 24

Chapter 3

Is The HCG Program Right For You?....................................... 27
    Endurance During Restrictive Stages 28
    Restrictions For Women... 28
    Financial Concerns.. 30
    Health Conditions That Will Hinder The HCG Diet Program 31
        Diabetes... 31
        Cancer 32
        Thyroid Problems 32
    Potential Side Effects That You Might Experience..................... 33
    Ascertain Your Health Condition First 34

Chapter 4

HCG Diet and Exercise: Is It Necessary To Go To The Gym? .. 35

Why The Common Exercise Routine Fail 36

How The HCG Approach Is Different 37

When Do You Start Exercising Normally Again 38

Chapter 5

How Much Pounds Should You Lose? 41

Check Your History 42

Body Mass Index (BMI) 44

Focusing On Your Size More 46

Chapter 6

Getting Started: The Right Preparation 47

Ask Professional Advice First 48

Look For HCG Supplies 49

Fill Up Your Fridge 50

Preparing For A Toxic-Free Lifestyle 52

Getting Rid Of Potential Hindrances 54

Recording Tools 54

Record Forms 55

Weekly Food Plan And Calorie Count 56

Daily Food Plan And Calorie Count 57

Monthly Weight Monitoring Table 58

Chapter 7

Common Mistakes You Need To Avoid 59

Learn everything about the program first 60

Always stick to the plan 60

Always bring a spare HCG supplement with you 61

Avoid Strenuous Physical Activities 62

Keep Those Questions Rolling 62

Make Sure Your HCG Supply Is Genuine 63

Conclusion 65

Introduction

Being obese has become very common in the US and no one can deny the fact that obesity is far too prevalent in other countries as well. The market for weight management products including diets, supplements, and weight programs have reached the new record of up to $150 Billion just a few years back.

It is a fact that people have always been wary of their own figure. They want to attain the golden numbers and become more attractive or more confident about themselves. But more than just the regular 'I want to look good' reason, there is also the matter of having a healthier body.

By shedding more pounds, people can experience a healthier lifestyle. They can avoid problems like heart failure, stroke, liver complications, and other medical problems related to being overweight and obese.

With all of these things that involve the weight of a person, it is not a surprise that people have continuously searched for ways to lose weight effectively. They went from diets, exercise routines, and even pills.

Along the history of weight loss, there have been many failures. Some showed good results but did not work for everyone. Also, there are those that posed health problems to the individual.

Lately however, there has been a buzz about a new weight loss program that promises fast and effective results. And more than just being effective, the program is also safe and did not pose serious health problems.

It is called the HCG weight loss program. In this book, you will learn everything you need to learn about it and how you can also shed extra pounds using the program.

So if you are overweight or if you look at the mirror and the person staring out at you looks fatter than you thought it should be, don't get disappointed just yet.

Chapter 1

HCG Diet: What Is It?

It is now the new craze in the world of weight loss and you may have already heard or read about it. Because of its growing popularity, it is now commonly on diet magazines, health websites, and other promotional channels. In fact, you may have already chanced by a news article saying that certain Hollywood celebrities are into the fad as well.

So with all these widespread propaganda seen on television, magazines, and the internet, you may ask, *what is HCG diet?* And more than just the question of what it really is, you may also be personally interested in the program. Perhaps you are looking for a brand new way to lose fat, something that will finally work?

In this book, everything that you need to know about the HCG program will be revealed to you in a step-by-step, detailed, and easy to understand manner. In addition, you will also be introduced to other important things that will help you along the way. So fasten your seatbelt because this is one ride towards better health and physique.

The HCG Program in General

To put it simply, the HCG program is an elaborate weight loss plan which utilizes a hormone called Human Chorionic Gonadotropin (HCG). Through controlled and well-planned intake of this naturally occurring hormone, the fat burning rate of the body is increased phenomenally. Other positive effects related to the hormone are also geared towards fat loss.

And in order to complement the effects of the hormone intake, the HCG program also includes an elaborate diet plan. Generally called the 'low calorie diet', this diet plan is designed to greatly boost the effects of HCG in the body. Together, HCG intake and low calorie diet will deliver positive results in a short time.

And unlike other weight loss programs which include an equally elaborate exercise plan, the HCG program excludes it. In fact, it is discouraged. Why this is so will be explained to you in greater detail in the succeeding chapters.

HCG: Where It Comes From

Alright, you might feel hesitant taking into your body something you are not familiar with, especially when the name is something like Human Chorionic Gonadotropin – not very easy to memorize is it not? But even though it is named complicatedly, it is actually safe and it occurs naturally in the body.

In nature, high levels of HCG can be found in the body of pregnant women. It is produced by the placenta and its production is at the highest rate during the earliest stages of pregnancy. The levels of HCG depletes as the pregnancy progresses into later stages until giving birth.

And although HCG is mostly associated with pregnancy, it is actually found in the body of all humans. It is not only present on gestating women or women in general but HCG can also be found in the body of men. So men who wish to lose body fat using the HCG program should have no fear.

The Dilemma of Fat:
The Good And The Bad

To make you appreciate better the HCG weight loss program, let us first take a look at some of the important matters that involve fat loss. While most people think that fat loss in general is a good thing in order to facilitate a drop in overall body weight, it is not always the case.

In more ways than one, severe fat loss is detrimental to health. Therefore, any person seeking ways to lose weight should pay close attention to the subject of fat loss. Losing fat is not always a good thing especially when done excessively.

When It Is Good

Fat loss is good when there is an excess of it. That means, you are taking in more than what your body needs and as a result, your body is storing it up in prone areas such as the belly, the arms, thighs, neck, and other areas.

Also, excessive fat gain can suffocate the internal organs as they get wrapped up in fat tissues. This situation makes it harder for organs to function properly. In situations such as this one, losing fat is generally healthy.

Other concern is the fact that additional fat tissues also require blood supply and nutrition. This means, the more body fat you are gaining, the more work there is for your circulatory system particularly the heart.

Some people also seek to lose fat for aesthetic reasons. There is nothing wrong with this because self-improvement can bestow confidence and self-esteem. However, the dieter must be careful not to lose more than what is necessary.

When It Is Bad

There is a reason why fat deposits exist in our body. During periods of time wherein our body is deprived of nutrition intake, these deposits serve as emergency energy. They are burned in order to compensate for the lack of food. Therefore, having a certain amount of fat in our body is healthy.

Fat also acts as a cushion for your joints, organs, and other crucial parts of your body. Without it, you will be more prone to injury. Losing these fats that help protect the body can result in a weaker body frame.

Also, there are certain fats that the body needs in order to function properly. Depriving your body of these fats can have detrimental effects on your overall health. So generally, fat loss is not good when it is done in excess.

Why Other Diet Programs Fail?

Because there are already far too many fat loss programs that precede the HCG program, you may think this is yet another one that will fail. But before you adapt that kind of thinking, examine first the following reasons why other programs fail:

Muscle Tissue Loss

Other programs do not care what you lose as long as your body exhibits weight loss. The problem is that some of those programs do not only result in fat loss but they also result in muscle loss. And when muscle loss in involved, the diet program will be short-lived and will soon fail. But why is this?

Maintaining muscle mass is important if you want to lose weight. The more lean muscle you have in your body, the greater is your body's capacity to burn fat. This is because lean muscles burn more fats than other tissues.

So even if your body experiences dramatic weight loss, all the lost weight will just return because your body also lost a lot of lean muscle mass. This is the cause of many rebounds, why some people lose weight and only gain them back after some time.

Intolerable Starvation

Many weight loss programs are accompanied by a controlled food intake. And even though there are weight loss programs that claim to include frequent food servings in order to avoid starvation, this is actually not the real case.

A diet plan may seem plentiful because it includes more five, six, or even seven meals a day. However, you will realize upon closer observation that each meal is less than a regular serving and is not enough to make you full. Also, most meals are not very appetizing or fulfilling.

So generally, a great majority of the weight loss programs out there will make you feel starved. And although this is something you can take for a few weeks or months, it is definitely not something anyone can maintain for longer periods of time. The diet will soon break and you will end up eating more servings again. This will result in a rebound.

Water Retention Loss

Also, many weight loss programs focus on preventing what is called 'water retention' – a phenomena wherein the body holds on to more fluid and results in greater body mass and bloated look.

However, focusing on water retention alone will not solve the problem in entirety because the fats will still be there. Also, prevention of water retention includes a specialize diet which is also hard to maintain. It can also lead to starvation and thus, a weight rebound.

Elaborate Exercise Programs

Do you know why people want to lose weight? Well, you may hear noble reasons like 'health improvement' but most of the time, it is about the looks. People want to look more beautiful and excess fat is making them feel frustrated and exhausted.

And imposing a tiring and time-consuming exercise program on these individuals will do any good. It will only make them more tired and more frustrated. It may work in the beginning, but people will soon start coming to gym less and less often. This plan is bound to fail sooner or later.

Why The HCG Diet Program Will Succeed

The HCG program gets right into the core of the problem. It targets excess body fats and burns it down without making the body lose lean muscle mass. As a result, you will only lose what you need to lose and it will be easier to maintain because your fat-burning muscles are still there.

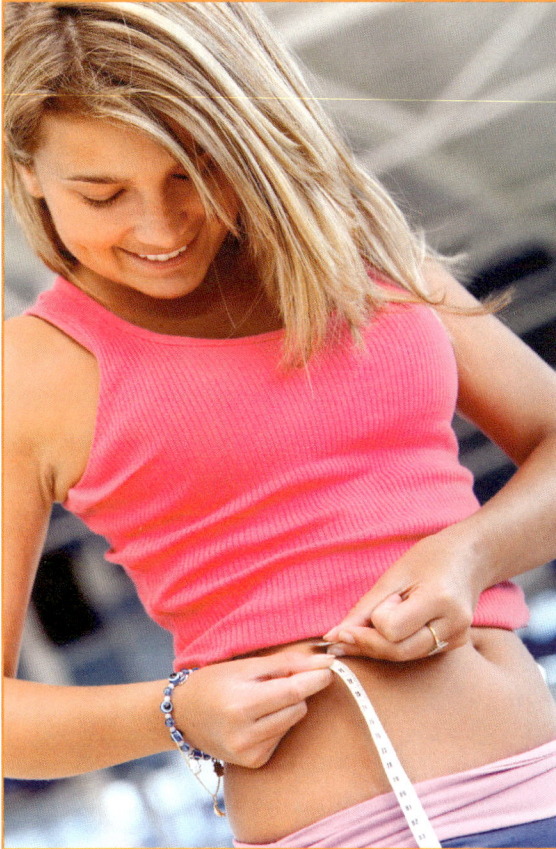

The problem of starvation is also solved easily. Yes, you may recall that the HCG program involves a low calorie intake but before you run away thinking that it will starve you, it is actually not the case. The HCG hormone you will be taking either orally or through injections will make you feel full and you will not feel starved at all.

Additionally, the HCG program will not impose upon you any laborious and time-consuming exercise program. Although regular exercise is always healthy, in the HCG program you should limit yourself to light exercises such as walking. All of this will be clear in the succeeding chapters.

Now that you know all the basics about the HCG weight loss program, it is time to introduce you into the program itself. In the next chapter, you will learn the phases that you will go through in the program.

Chapter 2:

The HCG Diet Plan: A Phase-By-Phase Approach

osing weight with the HCG weight loss program is a very rewarding experience because the results are easier to keep permanent. But if you really want it to work effectively for you, it is necessary to follow a straight guideline. This will avoid mistakes and rebounds.

The HCG weight loss program consists of three phases. The first phase focuses on preparing your body for the changes it will experience. In the next phase, the actual process or weight loss will begin. This is the time when you actually shed off those unwanted fat.

Lastly, the third phase is all about maintenance. It lowers down the restrictions present in phase two and is designed to maintain the results and keep the lost weight from coming back. If you need to lose more weight in the future, you can go back to phase one and redo the cycle.

Phase One:
Prepping Your Body

Phase one is designed to reset your body's metabolism and prepare it for the succeeding phases. It will only last for two days but because this step is what will set the stage for the amazing weight loss that is to follow, it is necessary to do things with close attention to every detail. Simply put, do it by the book.

But you will soon find that this phase is actually not hard to follow. During this stage, you are required to increase your intake of calories and fats. What that means for you is ramping up on all those foods that other diet programs want you to avoid. These may include chocolate cakes, chocolate bars, pork steak, beef stew, and others.

Quite appetizing is it not? Consider it as your temporary farewell to these great meals because the next step will mark the beginning of the low calorie and low fat diet. So rack up on your favorite meals and enjoy them for two days.

Also, phase one will mark the beginning of your HCG hormone intake. It does not matter whether you chose to take in orally or via injections. Either way, the amount and frequency of intake will be the same.

Another important guideline that you need to follow is the intake of at least 100 ounces of water every day. This will continue on throughout the succeeding phases. The reason for this is to increase the level of fluids within your body and allow better distribution of the HCG supplement.

Phase Two: Starting the Low Calorie Diet

Now here comes the most trying part of the cycle. The introduction of the low calorie diet may be difficult on most people especially that the first phase involved the intake of high calorie/high fat foods. However, the HCG hormone will help you along the way.

With the continuous intake of HCG hormone, your body will soon get used to the low calorie diet. This is because you will feel less hungry. Even though you are eating less, your body will not tell you that you are starving and your body will just continue to burn excess fat.

This is the beauty of the second phase. Other diet programs restrict your diet and crash your metabolism into starvation mode. As a result, your body will trigger irresistible hunger and force you to abandon the diet plan. But the HCG hormone will keep your metabolism up even during the low calorie diet.

So how much calorie should you limit to yourself during this phase? Throughout the second phase, you will be restricted to 500 calories per day. This number may scare you and natural instinct will tell you that it is not right. However, this phase will only last for 20 to 40 days.

Even though you are only eating 500 calorie worth of foods daily, your body will have all the energy it needs because the HCG supplement will burn down your excess fats. And during this period, you can begin losing weight at an incredible rate of up to two pounds per day.

So what do you eat while you are under such a very restricting calorie allowance? Some foods contain 500 calories per serving so you may wonder just what kind of foods you will be allowed to eat. To give you an idea, here is an example of what your daily diet will be like during the restrictive second phase:

- Two servings of fruit
- Two servings of vegetable
- One servings of lean meat

- Two melba toast
- Puree of one lemon

Other things that you must be careful of when serving these meals are high calorie additives. For example, you need to avoid salad dressings, oils, butter, garnishing such as grated cheese, and others.

If you must have flavor on your meals, restrict yourself to spices and herbs. For your drinks, it is okay to have coffee or tea but you must steer clear from creams. And while sugar is not allowed, you can have zero calorie sweeteners such as Stevia.

During this phase, you are also restricted from the intake of starchy carbohydrates such as breads. Now this may sound really hard to follow but the HCG supplement will help you not feel starved. Also, this phase is only temporary and most restrictions will be lifted when you enter the next phase.

Phase Three:
Entering the Maintenance Stage

Upon entering this stage, it can be assumed that you have already lost considerable body weight. If you underwent the second phase for 20 days, the expected weight loss is 15 pounds. If you did the maximum of 40 days, the loss of weight can be an amazing 40 pounds.

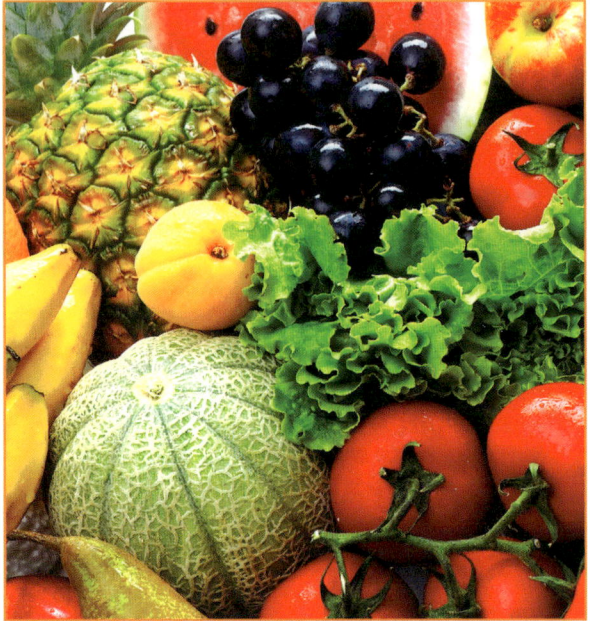

However, continuing on with the restrictive second phase is not healthy and that is why the third phase is developed. During this stage, most restrictions imposed by the second phase will be lifted gradually.

Please take note of the word "gradually" because this is crucial. Remember that you have been living on a 500 calorie diet during the last 20 or 40 days so your body will receive a shock if it immediately experiences a change in food intake.

So what you need to do is gradually increase your calorie intake until you reach the normal level which is less than 2000 calories in most adults. In any case however, you cannot start eating sugars and starches right away. You will have to wait around two to three weeks for these.

Some examples of starchy and sugary foods include: candy, rice, potatoes, cookies, bread, and cereals. Once you begin with these meals, start with smaller amounts and slowly increase the serving size to normal.

Curiously however, the third phase marks an increase in calorie and fat intake. You think that this will make you start gaining weight again. For other diet programs, that would be the case. But in HCG program, the effect is your metabolism will be corrected.

Re-entering the Cycle

A 15 pound from three weeks of low calorie diet or 40 pounds from six of it is very groundbreaking. However, there are those who might need to shed off more than just 15 or 40 pounds. In such cases, re-entering the cycle back to the first phase is possible.

In fact, entering the HCG program the second time around will help you lose more weight than you did the first time you entered the cycle. This is good news to people who want to lose more weight. With this, the ideal weight can be obtained in only a matter of months.

However, you cannot just re-enter the program anytime you want. At least, you need to put an allowance between cycles. When entering the program for the second time, a six weeks allowance is necessary. Here is a guideline for rest periods between cycles:

First cycle to second cycle   -   6 weeks rest

Second cycle to third cycle   -   8 weeks rest

Third cycle to fourth cycle   -   12 weeks rest

Fourth cycle to fifth cycle   -   20 weeks rest

Normally, it should only take a few cycles until you achieve your desired weight. In fact, having to take the HCG program up to the fifth time is quite rare. However, if you need to take a sixth cycle, you will have to wait for a period of six months.

Enjoying Permanent Changes

The second phase which is marked by a 20 to 40 days of low calorie and low fat intake will cause big changes within your body. After one cycle of the HCG program, you will realize that you no longer want the same things.

You will experience a new you. You are no longer hungry as often and you are no longer craving to overeat. However, these changes will not be permanent if you start your old eating habits again. Do not waste the changes that occurred in you and start living a healthy lifestyle.

Other than the changes in your cravings for food, you will also realize that your metabolism has improved. You are now more energetic and you can already last longer in physical activities. So you may want to include an exercise program into your schedule.

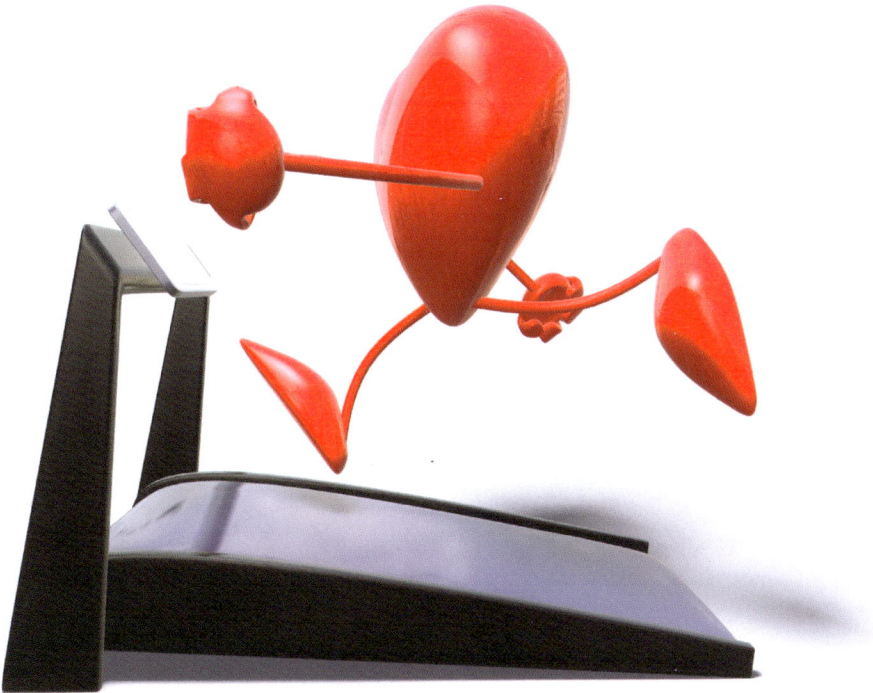

Chapter 3:

Is The HCG Program Right For You?

The HCG diet program allows you to experience big changes by starting big changes in your lifestyle, diet, and body chemistry. As such, it is only normal to assume that there are certain cases wherein the program might not be appropriate or safe.

In this book, you will learn the different situations and health conditions wherein the application of HCG diet program might become problematic. Study well these facts and use them to make a more sound decision whether the HCG diet is for you or not.

Lastly, if you fall under any of these conditions, you may want to consult a physician first if you are really intent on undergoing the program. Always remember that the administration of orally taken HCG hormone do not need prescription but is better taken under the supervision of a health professional.

Endurance during Restrictive Stages

If you read chapter two thoroughly, you are already aware of just how restrictive the HCG diet program can get especially during the second phase of the program. It especially makes restrictions on the food intake and lowers it down to 500 calories per day.

Also, if you chose to take HCG hormone via syringe shots, having to inject yourself regularly might become uncomfortable. And even if you chose to take the orally administered version, you still need to follow a strict guideline about intake.

All of these things that you need to follow during the course of the program will need discipline, endurance, and above all, accurate knowledge.

If you are not the type of person who is willing to devote time for these things, or if your lifestyle does not allow it, consider postponing the program until you are ready.

Restrictions for Women

There are several situations and conditions wherein a woman must not take part in the HCG diet program. One good example is in the case of pregnant women.

Take note that pregnant women need a specialized diet in order to properly sustain the nutritional needs of the baby in their womb. The restrictive diet of HCG program will hinder this to a great extent.

Also, women who are still in the stages of breastfeeding their child should not take part in the program. They too need a lot of nutrition in order to produce sufficient supply of nutritious milk. With the HCG diet, the milk producing capacity of their mammary glands will be hindered.

And even if you think you are not pregnant, but you are in the age or situation wherein pregnancy is highly likely, you should take a pregnancy test first before going through the HCG program. Many women fail to realize that they are pregnant during the earliest stages of pregnancy and you may mistakenly enter the program while you unknowingly are pregnant.

Also, if you are undergoing menopause stage and you are taking hormone replacements, the administration of additional hormone such as the HCG can hinder your treatment. It is best to avoid the HCG program during situations such as these.

If you are under any other medication, consult a physician first before undergoing the HCG diet program.

Financial Concerns

The HCG diet program is an effective method that will certainly help you shed off those extra pounds. However, the good results do come with a price tag. Although many people do not mind spending especially when it is about self-improvement and health, it cannot be dismissed that the financial demands of the program can become quite hectic for some.

Before undergoing the program, ascertain first if you can shoulder the financial demands. First, there is the HCG hormone supply. Whether you decided to take it by syringes or by homeopathic oral drops, there will be expenses involved. If you chose to take the hormone by injection, there will be extra expenses to maintain supplies like cotton balls, swabs, antiseptic wipes, syringe needles, and others.

Also, you might end up frequenting your physician during the program and physician's professional fees can be quite expensive. And the sad thing is that many health insurance companies do not cover HCG treatment.

So ask yourself first if you can or if you are willing to shoulder all of these expenses. If in the middle of the program you can no longer sustain the financial demands of the program, it will be troublesome to stop abruptly.

Health Conditions That Will Hinder the HCG Diet Program

Additionally, there are certain health problems that will not go well with the program. If you have a sickness or you are undergoing any medical treatment due to a health problem, you must ascertain first if the HCG program is safe for you. In any case, here are some situations that you need to be aware of:

Diabetes

So can diabetic people undergo the HCG program? The truth is that the HCG program can help improve the health condition of diabetic people. However, take note that it must be done under the strict supervision of a physician.

Diabetic patients are under a very strict diet code and they are also undergoing many treatments so the addition of the HCG program must be carefully super-vised. One reason is that the blood sugar must be contin-uously monitored.

But if the HCG program is properly integrated with the treatment of diabetic patients (only under the supervision of a physician), the associated weight loss can help improve the health condition. This is especially true for those with type II diabetes.

Cancer

Not to hit around the bush, the straight answer is: no you must not undergo the HCG diet program if 1) you currently have cancer, 2) you just recovered cancer treatment or 3) you have history of having cancer.

The reason is that the growth of cancer cells and tumors are linked to imbalances in the chemistry of hormones in the body. If you take HCG hormone into your bloodstream, it could worsen the situation.

Also, if you have abnormal growths which you suspect might be cancer, such as bumps around the breast area or if you have any irregularly shaped mole with varying surface color, consider avoiding the HCG treatment at the moment.

If you have symptoms and you have reasons to believe it might be cancer, ascertain your condition first with a physician before undergoing the HCG diet program.

But in all of these situations, if you are really intent on undergoing the HCG program you should consult your physician first. He might give it a go but only under certain situations. You must tread this path be carefully.

Thyroid Problems

Both hypothyroidism and hyperthyroidism are related to imbalances in the hormonal levels in the bloodstream.

Therefore, the administration of additional hormones into the body such as the HCG hormone can further upset situation. So for any health problem that involves the thyroid, it is best to avoid the HCG diet program.

However, it you really want to undergo the program because you do have some extra pounds to shed off, you can visit your physician and ask him if it is possible for you to undergo HCG treatment. If he gives it a go, it is best if he guides, monitors, and supervises you along the way.

Potential Side Effects That You Might Experience

Before we begin, you need to know that HCG supplement is not a diet drug. Therefore, you can expect less side effects compared to diet pills. Also, the drug is approved by the FDA (make sure you get one that is approved) so it is generally safe for public consumption.

However, it can be expected that there will be some effects. Check out first the side effects associated with HCG intake and determine if you are okay with them. Mostly, they will not really affect your lifestyle.

Here are some of the side effects that can be expected with HCG: head ache, increased heart rate and blood pressure, cramping, dizziness, nervousness, sleeping problems, gas, constipation, dry mouth, and diarrhea.

Ascertain Your Health Condition First

Additionally, it is possible that people are not even aware that they have a health problem. Many diseases and disorders do not manifest themselves in a way that is noticeable particularly during the earliest stages. Therefore, it is possible for you to undertake the HCG program unaware of your own health condition.

So even if you view yourself as a healthy person, it is still best to check with a physician if you are physically fit to undergo the HCG program. This will lessen potential problems in the future and ascertain the success of your weight loss plan.

Chapter 4:

HCG Diet And Exercise: Is It Necessary To Go To The Gym?

B ecause you are here reading this book, it is clear that you are a weightwatcher concerned with losing excess fat. If so, you may have already gone through many other weight loss methods. Looking back, you will notice they have something similar: they all include a rigorous exercise program.

In this chapter, you will discover how the HCG program is different. The programs allows for a safe and fast weight loss strategy without the inclusion of rigorous exercise – in fact, it will be restricted from you at some point along the phases of the program. Let us take this step by step and you will understand everything soon.

Why the Common Exercise Routine Fail

There is really nothing wrong with exercise and it is in fact a good thing. In fact, it is a universal truth that exercising will improve your health condition. But while this is true, do you think it is okay for a diabetic old woman to run 50 km as a professional marathon runner would?

The point here is that different people have different exercising needs. What is safe for one person given his situation may not be safe for others. Now what makes many weight loss programs fail is that they all demand a laborious exercise system.

Yes, there are people who can keep up with exercise programs like that, which is why there are success stories in those programs. But what if you are a regular employee, what if you are a housewife with children to care for, what if you simply do not have the time?

And even if you do have the time, majority of those who start out at gyms enthusiastically will soon lose the spirit. After all, who would want to keep doing the same thing over and over again for the rest of their lives? This is another reason why exercise programs fail. Few people can actually keep up with a laborious, tiring, and time-consuming routine.

Also, exercising can make you lose more than just fat. If it is not done correctly and not supervised by a professional, you could start losing lean muscle mass as well. As already explained in chapter one, this could lead to weight gain in the future.

How The HCG Approach Is Different

The HCG program does not encourage rigorous training – in fact, you are advised against it. This is

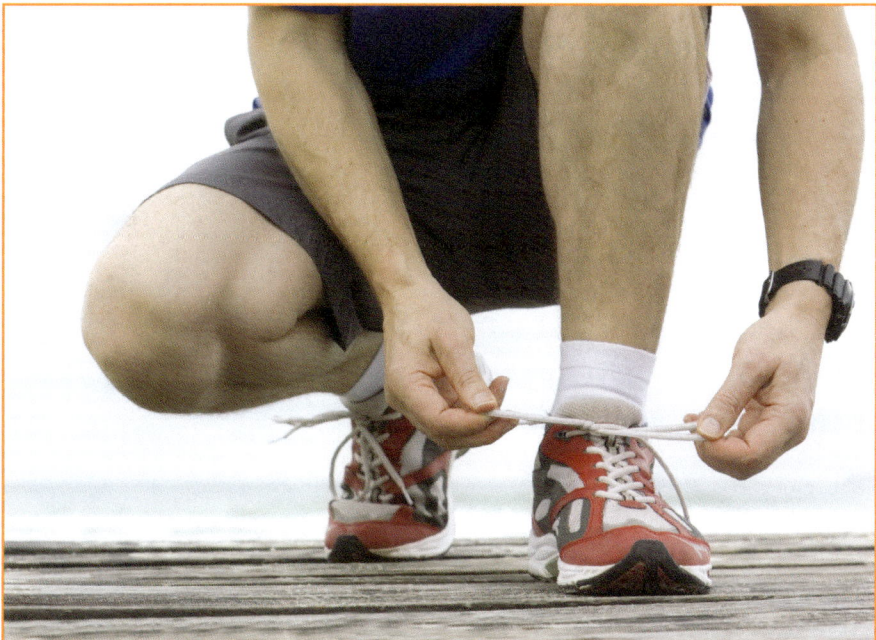

especially true during the second phase which is marked by a low calorie and low fat intake.

Since you are restricted to only 500 calories per day, exercising will force your body to burn more and you could end up exhausted. There is a possibility that you might go over the limit and collapse.

Now is that not good news? Finally, there is a weight loss program that advises against rigorous training in order to be effective. No longer will you have to endure long hours in the gym only to end up quitting a few weeks or months after.

But if you really must exercise just to keep your muscles in good condition, you should limit yourself to mild activities like walking. Also, it should not exceed 15 minutes. It should be enough to keep your blood pumping at a healthy rate. For flexibility exercises, you can go for light yoga, light stretching, and the sort.

If you insist on heavy exercises such as aerobics and weight gain, you can throw off the effects of HCG hormone supplements. As a response to the exercise, your body can switch to starvation mode. The entire plan will be hindered.

When Do You Start Exercising Normally Again

Once you are out of the restrictive secondary phase of the HCG program, you will enter the maintenance program which is less restrictive. Your diet will slowly be increased back to normal again and your energy rate may allow for more strenuous physical activities again.

As such, you may choose to start aerobics or weight training again. However, you must do it in a step-by-step manner. Gradually increase your capacity as you go along without taking things too fast. This is 'key' and you must abide by it.

But since it can be rather easy to overdo things if you start exercising on your own, here is clear guideline you can follow:

- Begin by prepping your body for the more strenuous exercises that will come in the following days or weeks. Walking and stretching would be a great idea. Do this for a couple more days until your body gets used to it.

- Instead of weight training, you first need to focus on improving the quality of your muscles. You can keep them lean with yoga exercises. With stretching, you can lengthen your muscle tissues and ready them for more exercises in the future.

- After a few days or a week of walking and stretching, you are now ready to add resistance training. But always remember to take things slowly from zero. Do not jump ahead to more difficult resistance training. Keep this for a few more days as you rev things up.

- After about two weeks of light exercises, you can begin with weight training again. This will improve your muscles and increase your body's capacity to naturally burn fat. Start with lightweights first. For men, a dumbbell with 2.5 kg plate on each side is appropriate enough. For women, a 2.5kg dumbbell is okay.

- And finally, you can spice things up by adding more adventurous physical activities such as hiking and canoeing. It really is up to. Find your interest and go on an adventure with your friends.

If you want to be just a bit more careful with everything, especially that you do not want anything to go wrong after undergoing the difficult phases of the HCG program, you may want to consult with a professional trainer. With supervision along the way, success will be closer.

Chapter 5:

How Much Pounds Should You Lose?

The HCG diet program will help you lose weight faster than any other method. However, you cannot keep shedding off pounds continuously. At some point, you will reach your desired figure and halt the weight loss. But the big question is, when?

Truth be told, many weightwatchers do not know when to stop. They become so obsessed with weight loss that they fail to realize they have already reached their desired weight. As a result, they face another set of problems – malnutrition and being underweight.

There is also the danger of anorexia – a disorder marked by an incessant obsession to dieting regardless of the subject's bony structure and continuously dropping weight. This condition can be serious and can result in many health problems.

Another potential problem is that people might impose upon themselves too high a goal. When the goal is too high, there is a high possibility that it will not be achieved, or at least, that it will not be achieved soon enough.

As a result of failure due to excessive goals, frustration can step in. This can hinder the weight loss and a rebound can result in the process. Therefore, you must avoid all of these tendencies.

Once way you can do this is to set the "right goal". You have to know just how much weight is okay for you to lose. Additionally, you also need to be realistic about the length of time frame that you can achieve this goal. You should also be ready for potential extensions should you not achieve it in time.

Basically though, there is really no telling exactly how much weight your body can lose. However, there are methods you can use to get the approximate figures. Here are some ways that can help:

Check Your History

Most people do not maintain the same physique all throughout their lives. There are times when they are overweight, times when they are underweight, and times when they are at their best figure. And by looking at your body's history, you can tell what figure your body is capable of supporting or how far it can go in terms of weight loss.

For example, you can ask questions like, *have I always been overweight and large?* In such cases, perhaps your body is designed to have a larger frame and there is a limit to just how much weight you can actually lose. If you are in this situation, it may be wiser to set lower goals.

This is of course not to say that you will never reach the figure you dream of. It is possible but it may be better to take things slowly. For example, if you are 200 pounds and you have always been in the extra large department since childhood, you should not aim to lose 80 pounds straight away.

In the beginning, you can aim for 20 pounds. After achieving that, goal, aim for another 20 pounds and so forth. This will avoid frustrations and make your task seem easier than it really is.

Also, dividing your bigger goal into several smaller ones will harmonize with the design of the HCG weight loss program. Going back to chapter 2, the weight loss part which is the second phase of the program should be taken with time spaces in between. So you can lose some in the first cycle and lose more in the following cycles.

So how can you establish a history check of your previous figures? Well, you cannot really expect to pull out a record of your weight history since childhood so what you need to do is check the photo albums.

Get as many photographs as you can from all stages of your life. When you do, you just have to make an estimate of how much you weigh at each given point in time. You do not need to be specific because the only thing you really need is to establish a pattern.

Body Mass Index (BMI)

The body mass index is a simple number derived from a rather complicated formula. What the body index represents is the value which determines if you are overweight, underweight, or normal.

For beginners, here is a guideline about what the numbers would represent and what it means for your body health:

- BMI Value 18 to 25 – Normal
- BMI Value 25 to 30 – Overweight
- BMI Value 30 above – Obese
- BMI Value below 18 – Underweight

So how do you arrive at the values? There is really no need for you to memorize the formula. Besides, doing the math yourself could result in human error and you could wind up with the wrong figure.

For a more reliable computation of your Body Mass Index, you can turn to the internet and search for BMI calculators. All that you need to input is your height and weight. Nowadays, it should be rather easy and simple to find calculators that calculate BMI.

However, the value represented by BMI calculators is not absolute. Always remember that there is always more to your figure that just your weight and height. A person can have a BMI value of above 25 but is healthier and more figure perfect than someone with a BMI value of less than 25.

When factoring your BMI value into your decision of how much weight to lose, only use it as a reference and not as an absolute fact. It will give you an idea of how much you need to lose.

In any case, if your BMI value represents an unhealthy figure of above 25, you can try inputting into the calculator a lower weight value. Keep testing until you come up with a less than 25 BMI number. Whatever is the difference between your actual weight and the false weight number that produced a healthy BMI number should be the weight you need to lose.

Focusing On Your Size More

In many situations, your weight may not be the only factor that you need to watch. It is very possible that you may have already attained a picture perfect figure even though the scales are still showing a higher than normal weight value.

For example, you may have set a goal to achieve a weight of only 120 pounds. But it may happen that even though you only lost enough weight to be around 140 pounds, your size may already be golden.

How is this possible? Actually, people of the same measurements can weigh differently. This is because other factors are at work. Maybe the other person has more muscle mass and the other has more fat tissue mass (lean muscle and fat weigh differently).

Also, there is the bone mass. The heavier person may simply have a higher bone density than the lighter person. But if you look at them side by side, they look about the same in size.

So do not just focus on your weight but also watch your size and body measurements. Even if your weight is still more than what you aimed for, losing more can make you look too thin.

Chapter 6:

Getting Started: The Right Preparation

Before you go out on a picnic, you plan ahead of time and get the things you need ready. If you jump into the activity right away, you can forget things and everything can become un-successful. The same goes when you enter a weight loss diet program.

With the HCG diet loss program, you have to be prepared ahead of time. There are supplies that you need to take care of, and you also need to set yourself at the right mental state. This will help you along the way and keep the program stable.

But of course, it will just be as much of a mess if you try to do things at the same time. For a step-by-step procedure, here is a list of things that you need to take care of before entering the program. It is listed in sequence so you will not get lost along the way.

Ask Professional Advice First

It is never right to make changes in your body's system without the supervision of a knowledgeable professional. Before entering the HCG diet program, consider visiting a doctor first. Your family doctor should be a good idea because he knows your medical background.

For women, you should check first of you are pregnant. You need to make sure that you are not. Also, consider several contraceptive methods right after entering the program. You will not want to become pregnant during the course of the HCG diet program.

You should also check for diabetes, cancer, or abnormal growths that could eventually develop into cancer. Even if you do not have cancer, growths like cancerous moles can develop faster into cancer because of the HCG hormone supplements.

It is a lot better if you manage to find a doctor who has experience in attending to patients that undergo HCG diet program. If you have friends or colleagues also undergoing the program, as them which doctor is attending to them or if they have any recommendations.

Also, keep in mind that you are not only looking for a professional who will determine whether you are physically fit for the program or not. You are also looking for someone who will monitor your progress and keep watch of you as you go along with the program. This will avoid accidents.

Look For HCG Supplies

For beginners or for those who are entering the HCG diet program for the first time, it is best to go for a beginner's kit. Usually, a single kit is good enough for one cycle. This means, you will not run out of supply until you finish an entire cycle and will not be hindered.

Also, starter's kits usually come with a guideline or manual book which determines proper intake procedures, dosages, and other concerns. Make sure to read them carefully. Just as a precaution though, if you can afford it, but two sets. Leave one at home and take the other one with you all the time. This way, you will always have HCG supplements wherever you go and not miss an intake.

Usually, starter's kits are in the form of homeopathic or orally taken HCG. This is good for beginners. But if you choose to go for syringe shots, you will need a prescription write up from your doctor.

In both cases, whether you are going for injections or homeopathic drops, make sure that you buy enough supplies for at least one cycle. Also, know all the nearby shops that sell them. Ask the pharmacist if they often run out of supplies. If they do, stock up and be familiar with other sellers of the supplement.

Fill Up Your Fridge

If you recall from chapter two, the first, second, and third phase of the program all have different dietary needs. During the first phase, you are required to undergo a high calorie and high fat diet. Next, you will enter a restrictive low calorie diet. For the last or maintenance phase, you will again slowly regain your normal diet.

So what do all of these mean for you? It means of course than you will need to stock up on the necessary foods. If you do not, you could wind up eating the wrong sorts. This can have adverse effects on the program if you eat the wrong foods. As a guideline, here are the foods that you will need to have in the fridge:

- **Fresh fruits to ensure rich vitamin supply**. This is important to facilitate better bodily functions during the changes that you will experience.

- **Lemons**. You will make juices out of these to make your drinks more exciting. This will make it easier to endure a low calorie diet. Match it up with a zero-calorie sweetener to make it more appetizing.

- **Fresh vegetables.** For a supply of fiber and necessary nutrients throughout the program. Fibers will also help maintain better digestive activity especially during the phase wherein you restrict your food intake.

- **Lean meats.** These can be chicken meat or fish meat. Occasionally, you can also have lean beef and pork meats. These will give life to your diet and provide the necessary protein supply.

- **Coffee and tea.** Your diet is already restricted enough so it will be even more difficult to endure if you reduce the variety of your drinks. Coffee and tea will help you along the way and also provide a rich source of antioxidants.

- **Fat free dairy products.** Stock up on fat free yogurt to satisfy your sweet tooth. Also, you can have fat free cottage cheese.

- Additionally, you might want to make each meal extra special considering that you are restricted to a 500 calorie diet during the second phase of the program. To make every meal more appetizing, here are some safe add-ons you can have:

- Paprika

- Cinnamon

- Pepper

- Parsley

- Low fat seasonings

And for very trying moments that you are really craving for something more than just your regular restrictive diet plan, here are some foods you can indulge on:

- Cinnamon Apple Crunch

- Berry Sobet

- Fruit Smoothie

- Cinnamon Toast

- Stevia zero-calorie artificial sweetener

Preparing For A Toxic-Free Lifestyle

The HCG diet program involves the intake or injection of the hormone called Human Chorionic Gonadotropin. To make it work at its best, you should avoid foods that contain ingredients that affect hormonal activities. Foods that have plenty of these ingredients are those not produced naturally.

So while you are undergoing the HCG diet program, you should invest on buying only organic foods. Here is a quick guideline about organic foods and what the labels mean:

- 100% Organic. If you see this, it means that the product as a whole is made up of only natural ingredients.

- Organic Food. If you only see the label 'Organic' without the term '100%', it means the product is at least 95% made of only natural ingredients.

- Made of organic ingredients. When this is on the label, only a good 70% or the product is made up of organic materials.

For your HCG diet program, you will only want to stock up on the first two. You can only go for the third one if there is no other alternative.

Another thing that you want to avoid is cosmetics. These may include lotions, face creams, and makeup. Take note that although these products are applied topically, some of their components are absorbed by the body and make it to the bloodstream.

Of course, you can still have lotions, creams, and light makeup. But go for those that are organic. Yes, the organic label is not only found on foods but also on cosmetics and even furniture.

Getting Rid Of Potential Hindrances

If you are here reading this book, chances are that you have some pounds to shed off. This may also mean that your current kitchen is a house of temptations. There could be canned goods, hams, pastas, chocolate bars, and other high calorie and high fat foods.

Before entering the program, consider getting rid of these things first. Well, it may be a waste to just throw all of them away. So as an alternative, you box them up, seal them in a way that it will difficult for you to re-open them, and place them on the attic or storage room.

If the food will spoil soon, just consider giving it away. Maybe give it as a gift to relatives or neighbors. They will be more than happy to have them.

Recording Tools

The HCG diet program is composed of phases and stages. Therefore, it is a good idea to record your achievements along the way. It will make it easier for you to track how well you are doing or if there is something that you are not doing right.

Here are things that you will need:

- Notebook or journal

- Pens

- Weight scale

- Measuring tape

So what will you record? It depends on what you need to keep track of. Maybe you want to list down the calorie count of every food you eat so you know if you are already going above your set limit.

Also, you have to record the changes in your weight as well as the changes in your body measures. It will serve as a good reference for the future. You also need to keep record of your HCG supplement intake.

Food menus, recipes, eating schedule, and shopping lists are just some of the other things that you need to keep track of.

Record Forms

Additionally, you might want to be extra organized with how you take note of things. Here are some sample forms that you can use:

Weekly Food Plan And Calorie Count

	Mon	Tues	Wed	Thurs	Fri	Sat	Sun
Breakfast Calorie Value							
Lunch Calorie Value							
Dinner Calorie Value							
Snack Calorie Value							

Daily Food Plan And Calorie Count

	Food List	Calorie Value	
Breakfast	• • •		
Lunch	• • •		
Dinner	• • •		
Snack	• • •		

Monthly Weight Monitoring Table

	Week 1	Week 2	Week 3	Week 5	Week 5
Upper Arm					
Thigh					
Waist					
Bust/Chest					
Hips					

Chapter 7:

Common Mistakes You Need To Avoid

Up until now you learned how to make the HCG program work wonders for you. Of course, there will be a lot of effort on your part to make is successful but all of those efforts will be rewarded. You will have a better figure and a better health.

But knowing all the right things is only one side of the whole story. To help you avoid the pitfalls, you need to know where they are. This mans, you need to know the common mistakes that makes the HCG diet program ineffective.

In this chapter, you will be informed about the mistakes that can throw off the entire plan. Know them and learn from them.

Learn everything about the program first

One common mistake that people do is that they just jump right into the program without really knowing anything. If you have read everything from chapter one up until here and did every requirement mentioned, it can be said that you are now knowledgeable enough.

Some people however are blinded by the idea of quick weight loss. They take the program and just expect to learn things along the way. This is detrimental. As you have learned so far, it is essential to plan ahead.

Read books about the program (this one is already covered by this book), know the places where you will be buying the supplies, know the availability, check with your physician, know your health condition, and check with your financial stability.

Always stick to the plan

The ways and the methods of the HCG program are unconventional. Just imagine, you will be restricted to a low 500 calorie diet and you will be restricted from strenuous physical activities. As a result, some people may feel the need to change some things.

Rest assured however that everything within the HCG diet program has a reason. If you change anything, it could have a domino effect and affect the entire program. Stay with the book instructions and heed the warnings and instructions of the physician that monitors you during the program.

Always bring a spare HCG supplement with you

One of the most important points of the program is to take the hormone regularly and on time. And sadly, there are many situations that might avoid you from following this crucial instruction.

For example, you may be out of the office by 5:00 PM and you expect to be home at 7:00 PM – just in time for your 7:00 PM shot of HCG. But what if you got caught in a long traffic along the way, or maybe there is an emergency work that you need to attend to.

On situations like that one, it is always best to have a spare HCG supplement with you all the time. You cannot let unexpected things ruin the program because it will also ruin your plans of successfully losing weight.

Avoid Strenuous Physical Activities

The norm of the society says that maintaining a healthy exercise routine composed of aerobics and occasional weight-lifting is necessary in order to lose or maintain weight. You should not let this norm confuse you.

Yes, you will also do these kinds of exercises but not too soon. During the early stages of the program, you will need to avoid it. If you engage in such strenuous activities, your body will enter starvation mode and the HCG will be ineffective.

As a result of the starvation mode, your body will slow down the rate at which it burns fat, it will make you feel hungry, and you will absorb more of the food that you will eat. This is not something you want to happen.

Keep Those Questions Rolling

When you are new to something, it is normal that there are many things you do not understand. This can be true even after reading plenty of books and online tutorials. So what you need to do is keep those questions rolling.

Some people fear asking because they do not want to bother others or they do not want to look ignorant. This is a big mistake. Your doctor should always be happy to answer inquiries. Ask questions so you will not end up with guess work and mess everything up.

Make Sure Your HCG Supply Is Genuine

Now, the last thing you want to happen is end up with a fake HCG supplement. Not only are these ineffective, but they can also pose many health problems. This could lead to terrible accidents.

And even if the supplement genuinely contains HCG, it may not be properly manufactured so it can still be considered fake. Make sure that you buy only products manufactured by United States pharmaceutical companies. Also, look for the FDA approval seal.

If you find anything that is too cheap, that is one reason to suspect. Also, it is best to avoid shopping online for HCG. If you will be buying online, only go for trusted and reputable sources.

For other concerns, you may want to speak with your doctor. They will know best what you should avoid, what you need to watch out for, and what you need to do and how to do them correctly.

Conclusion

The HCG weight loss program is an effective method to lose weight and many people have already benefitted from it. And because it is designed to help you keep those pounds from coming back, it is easier to maintain the healthier figure you will attain.

However, you need to keep in mind that the effectiveness of the program will depend on you. The HCG program can give you the body you have been dreaming of but you need to work hard to keep it that way.

Discipline is necessary. By focusing on your goals, you can keep the lost pounds from coming back. You will live a healthier life and you will also gain confidence in just about everything.

You also need to acknowledge that having a better figure is not all there is to being more attractive. You also need to watch the way you wear clothes and the way you treat other people.

So instead of just focusing on the diet, you also need to improve your character and your selection of clothes. Be wary that you will lose a lot of pounds with the HCG weight loss program so better be ready to shop for new clothes.